—THE— Fast Diet Recipe Book

THE Fast Diet Recipe Book

New and Improved

Healthy Weight Loss and Low Calorie Fast Diet Recipes

GILLIAN HYMAN

Copyright © 2013 Gillian Hyman

The Fast Diet Recipe Book
Vineyard Publishing
All Rights Reserved

No part of this publication may be reproduced, stored in a retrieval system or transmitted, in any form or by any means, electronic, mechanical, photocopying, recording or otherwise, without proper written permission from the author. The only exception is a reviewer. A reviewer may quote brief passages in a review.

ISBN-13: 978-1493676774

Printed in the United States of America

~ Table of Contents ~

A SCIENTIFIC WEIGHT LOSS SUCCESS – THE FASTDIET 9

FAST DIET BREAKFAST UNDER 200 CALORIES 11

    Strawberry Banana Pancakes 11

    Hearty Breakfast Bowl 14

    Sizzling Fruit Pockets 16

    Chives Scrambled Eggs 18

    Easy Poached Egg 20

    Tortilla Delight 22

    Quick Kipper Fillet 25

    Berry Smoothie 27

    Healthy Blueberry Pancakes 29

    Tasty Baked Veggies 31

    Guilt-Free Egg Sandwich 33

    Peachy Citrus Smoothie 35

    Cheddar & Beans Omelet 37

    Raspberry Banana Smoothie 39

FAST DIET LUNCH & DINNERS UNDER 250 CALORIES 41

    Holiday Zesty Honey Gammon 41

    Italian Seasoned Red Potato 44

Mustard Turkey Cottage 46

Easy Chili Scallops 48

Porky Chestnut Stew 50

Beefy Barbeque Lettuce Wraps 52

Herb Baked Cod 54

Sweet 'n' Spicy Salmon 56

Spicy Turkey Cooked Vegetables 58

Vegan Creamed Tortilla Wraps 60

Fish 'n' Veggie Tacos 62

Squash Zucchini Split 64

Turkey Zucchini Bolognese 66

Veggie Chicken Mix 68

Sweet Turkey Pepper Bowl 70

Deluxe Thai Salad 72

Avocado Tortilla Chowder 74

Spicy Vegetable Bowl 76

Asian Style Chicken Salad 78

Creamy Orange Carrot Soup 80

Lemon Smoked Salmon 82

Minty Green Pea Soup 84

Delicious Vegan Coleslaw 87

Olive Baked Potatoes 89

Tasty Vegetable Delight 91

Healthy Mashed Potatoes... 93

Tomato and Kale Soup... 95

Lemon Beetroot Salad... 97

Spicy Prawn Soup 99

Red & Green Ham Salad... 101

Healthy Spring Vegetable Soup.. 103

Special Beetroot and Bramley Soup 105

Carrot Lentil Soup... 107

Quick & Easy Asparagus and Salmon 109

Flavourful Lemon Grilled Chicken Breast................................. 111

Tasty Grilled Sea Bass 113

Chicken Salad 115

You Can Do It!... 117

Disclaimer

The information provided in this book is for educational purposes only. I am not a physician and this is not to be taken as medical advice or a recommendation to stop eating other foods. The information provided in this book is based on Dr. Michael Mosley Fast Diet research and recommendations. You should consult your physician to ensure that the recipes in this book are appropriate for your individual circumstances. If you have any health issues or pre-existing conditions, please consult your doctor before implementing any of the Fast Diet recipes presented in this book. Cooking results may vary from individual to individual. This book is for informational purposes only and the author does not accept any responsibilities for any liabilities or damages, real or perceived, resulting from the use of this information.

A Scientific Weight Loss Success – The FastDiet

In the latter part of 2012, Dr. Michael Mosley revealed his scientifically tested findings about the power of intermittent fasting (IF). It is important to note that intermittent fasting is also known as the Fast Diet or the 5 2 Diet. In his book, The FastDiet, doctor Mosley addressed the flaws involved in low–fat diets or exercise programs which NEVER suggested skipping a meal! Consequently, it is no wonder that most people have problems with their weight and health.

Along with Doctor Mosley, National Columnist, Mimi Spencer also added to the dynamism of the whole Fast Diet concept by providing helpful and practical means of safely following through on an intermittent Fasting Diet.

Based on biblical and scientific evidence, as well as personal experience, Dr. Mosley along with other medical experts have come to agree that our bodies were designed for intermittent fasting.

How does Dr. Michael Mosley's FastDiet really work?

According to Dr. Mosley, the fast diet involves partial fasting (eating really light) for two non-consecutive days per week. In addition, this thoroughly researched and tested diet has a few gender specific factors. Men are permitted a maximum caloric intake of 600 calories on the days of fasting, while women are permitted a caloric intake of no more than 500 calories on those two fasting days. Plenty of water is best on Fast Days and if you really want some flavor, you can opt for herbal tea, green tea, black tea and even black coffee. Guess what's liberating? On the other days of the week, men or women are permitted to eat WHATEVER they want! With a resounding "yes", this strategy has worked effectively for Dr. Mosley and countless others around the world.

Consequently, this profound diet plan has accounted for the popularity of Dr. Mosley's Book, *FastDiet*.

As with any adaption to a new diet, it is always handy to have several meal options close at hand. This is why having tried the FastDiet, I have decided to share these interesting Fast Diet recipes with you. Fasting days can be challenging, so why not make your life easier?

In this FastDiet Recipe Book you'll find healthy, tasty, balanced and calorie-counted meals. Now, you can lose weight and live healthy the easy way. Get ready, you can do it!

FAST DIET BREAKFAST UNDER 200 CALORIES

Strawberry Banana Pancakes

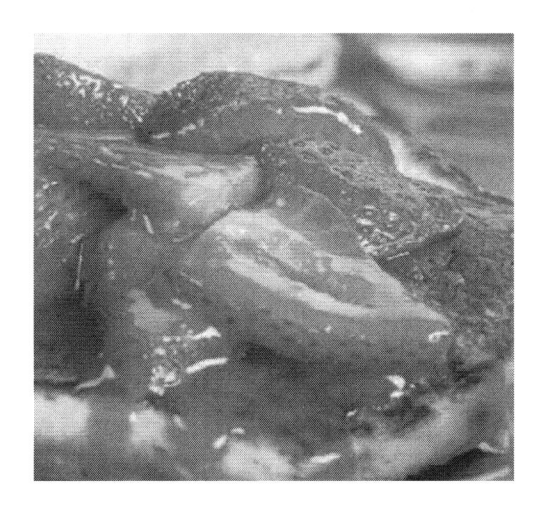

Cooking Minutes: *10 minutes*

Preparation Time: *10 minutes*

Calorie per Serving: *109 Calories*

Makes 2 Servings *(2 pancakes per serving)*

Ingredients:

½ of a large Banana, peeled and sliced

½ cup (118 grams) Whole Wheat Pancake Mix

¼ cup (60 ml) Water

Flora Cooking Spray

Topping:

½ cup (118 grams) of Frozen Strawberries, thawed and sliced

1 tablespoon (15 ml) Orange Juice

Directions:

1. Put the banana in a medium bowl and puree with fork.
2. Add the pancake mix and water and mix all ingredients.
3. Spray a large skillet with flora cooking spray and heat to medium heat.
4. Add ¼ cup batter for each pancake into hot skillet. Cook the pancakes completely on the two sides for about 2 minutes on each side of the pancake.

Topping Directions:

1. To make the topping, spray a skillet with cooking spray and heat over medium heat.
2. Cook strawberries and orange juice for 3 minutes or until the berries are soft.
3. Use a spoon to add the topping to pancakes and serve.

Hearty Breakfast Bowl

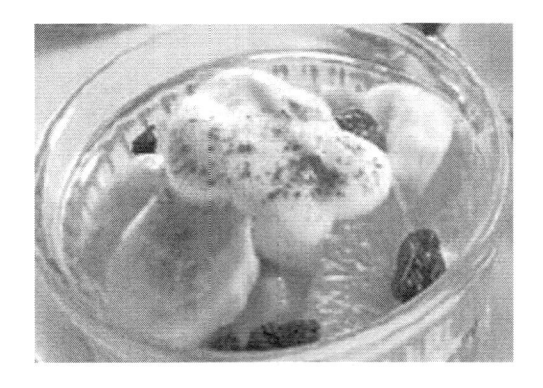

Cooking Minutes: *None*

Preparation Time: *5 minutes*

Calorie per Serving: *81 Calories*

Makes 2 Servings (1/2 cup per serving)

Ingredients:

1 Orange, peeled, pitted, and chopped

½ of a medium Banana, peeled and sliced

½ tablespoon (8 grams) Raisins

2 tablespoons (30 ml) Vanilla Yogurt - low fat

¼ teaspoon Ground Cinnamon

Directions:

1. Combine fruits in a bowl small.
2. Equally divide fruits for 2 bowls.
3. Add to the fruit one heaping tablespoon low-fat yogurt, and sprinkle some cinnamon before serving.

Sizzling Fruit Pockets

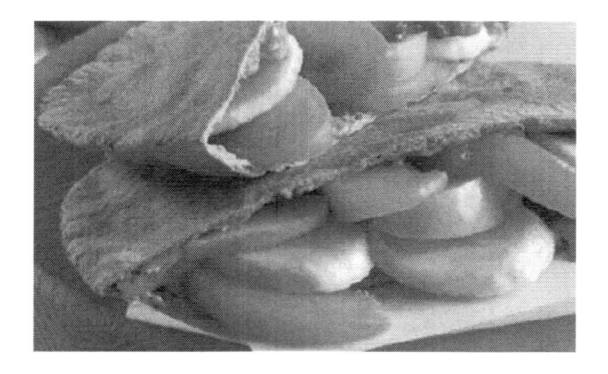

Cooking Time: *10 seconds*

Preparation Time: *10 minutes*

Calorie per Serving: *180 Calories*

Makes 2 Servings *(½ pita pocket per serving)*

Ingredients:

1 Whole Wheat Pita Loaf

1/8 cup (30 ml / 30 grams) Peanut Butter, low-fat

¼ of an Apple, seeds and core removed, cut into thin slices

¼ of a Banana cut into thin slices

¼ of a Fresh Peach, thinly sliced

Directions:

1. Cut pita loaf in half to make 2 pockets. Heat them in the microwave for about 10 seconds to soften.
2. Carefully open each pocket and brush the interior walls with a thin layer of peanut butter.
3. Fill the pockets with a mixture of apple slices, banana and peach. Serve at room temperature.

Chives Scrambled Eggs

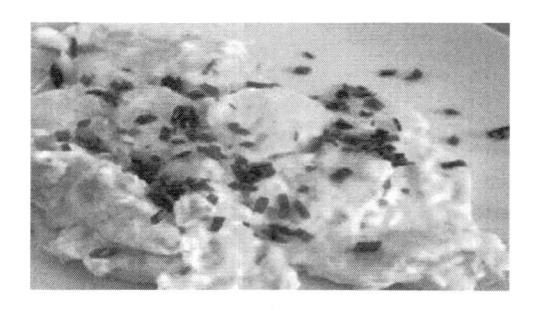

Cooking Minutes: *3-5 minutes*

Preparation Time: *15 minutes*

Calorie per Serving: *92 Calories*

Makes 2 Servings

Ingredients:

Flora Cooking Spray

2 large Eggs

½ cup Egg whites

1 tablespoon Fresh Chives, chopped

¼ teaspoon coarse Kosher Salt (more will be needed for sprinkling)

Pepper to taste

Directions:

1. In a medium bowl, whisk eggs, egg whites, chopped chives, and ¼ teaspoon salt until well blended.
2. Heat a heavy medium nonstick skillet over medium heat. Coat with Flora Cooking Spray, add eggs and stir with heatproof silicone spatula until eggs are almost cooked but still partly runny, tilting nonstick skillet while mixing with a spatula so that the uncooked portion runs underneath, approximately 2 minutes. Take from heat.
3. Add additional sprinkle of kosher salt and pepper as needed. Top with whole chives, if you so desire.

Easy Poached Egg

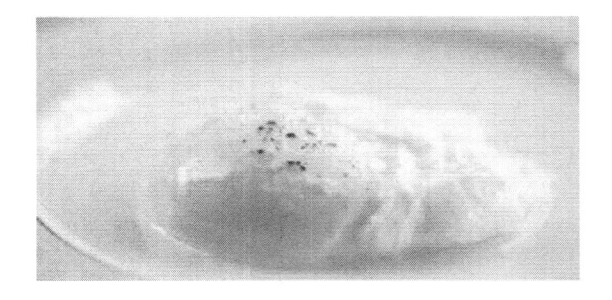

Cooking Minutes: *1-3 minutes*

Preparation Time: *1 minute*

Calorie per Serving: *74 Calories*

Makes 1 Serving

Ingredients:

1 large Egg

1/3 cup (78 ml) water

Salt and Pepper to taste

1/8 teaspoon White Vinegar

Directions:

1. In a 6 ounce custard cup, add the water and white

vinegar. Break egg into cup, pierce egg yolk with toothpick, and cover dish loosely with microwave safe plastic wrap. Place in microwave and cook for about a minute or until according to your preference.

2. Cooking times may vary based on the wattage of your microwave and taste preference.

3. Immediately remove egg from hot water with a slotted spoon. Add salt and pepper to taste for serving.

Tortilla Delight

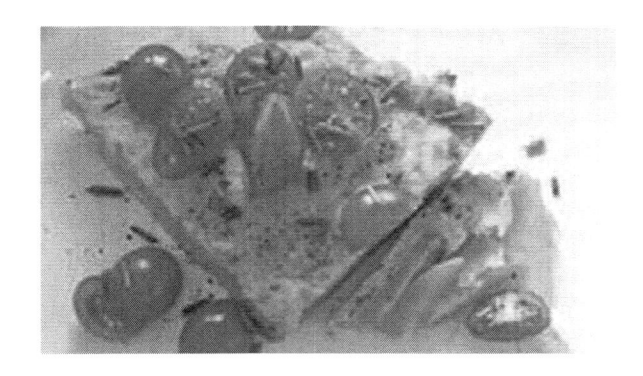

Cooking Minutes: *35 minutes*

Preparation Time: *15 minutes*

Calorie per Serving: *190 Calories*

Makes 4 Servings

Ingredients:

1 medium Yukon Gold Potato (about ½ pound/226 grams)

1 large Egg White

1 tablespoon Olive Oil

1 Garlic Clove, minced

3 tablespoons Manchego Cheese, finely grated

1 teaspoon Extra-Virgin Olive Oil

½ cup halved Grape or Cherry Tomatoes

1 tablespoon minced and divided Fresh Chives

¾ teaspoon Salt, divided

½ teaspoons Freshly Ground Black Pepper

4 large Eggs

½ cup (about ½ pound/226 grams) Halved Grape or Cherry Tomatoes

Directions:

1. Preheat oven to 350 degrees Fahrenheit.
2. Place Yukon Gold potato in a saucepan or pot and pour enough water to cover the potatoes and bring to boiling point. Lower heat, and allow to simmer for about 20 minutes or until properly cooked. Drain potato, cool and peel it, then make thin slice.
3. Add 2 teaspoons chives, salt, pepper, eggs, and egg white in a bowl. Stir with a whisk until fully blended.
4. Heat 1 tablespoon oil in an 8-inch ovenproof nonstick skillet on medium heat. Add in minced garlic and potatoes slices then cook for about 30 seconds while turning the potato gently in order to coat it with oil. Add in the remaining salt by sprinkling.
5. Press potato mixture with a spatula into a solid layer in bottom of pan. Add in the mixture with the egg over the potato mixture and cook for about a minute. Slowly mix the egg mixture with the potato mixture.
6. Press potato back down in bottom of pan and allow to

cook for about 2 minutes. Take from heat. Evenly add grated cheese.

7. Bake for approximately 7 minutes or until center is firm. Take from oven. Sprinkle with a teaspoon of extra-virgin olive oil. Set the sides of tortilla loose from the pan then gently place it on a serving plate. Add the tomatoes and remaining chives.

Quick Kipper Fillet

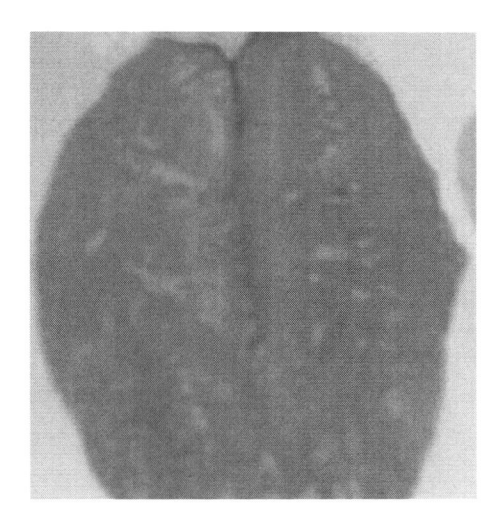

Cooking Minutes: *3-5 minutes*

Preparation Time: *5 minutes*

Calorie per Serving: *140 Calories*

Makes 1 Serving

Ingredients:

1 Kipper Fillet

1 teaspoon Olive Oil

2 tablespoon Fresh Parsley, chopped (optional)

½ teaspoon Lemon Juice

Salt and pepper to taste

Directions:

1. Place Kipper fillet in a microwave safe dish.
2. Drizzle over olive oil, parsley, lemon juice, salt and pepper. Cover with microwave safe Cling Film for 2½ to 3 minutes.
3. Serve and enjoy. This can be served with wilted spinach and a poached egg for breakfast.

Berry Smoothie

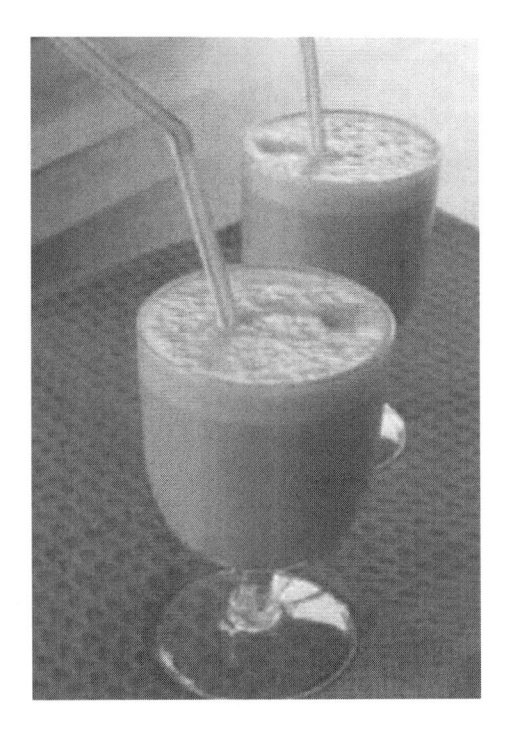

Preparation Time: *10 to 12 minutes*

Calories per Serving: *100 Calories*

Makes 4 Servings

Ingredients:

100 ml (about 1/2 cup) Low-Fat Cow's Milk

200 ml (about ¾ cup) Natural Yogurt

250 ml (1 cup) Cranberry Juice

175 grams (6.2 ounces) Frozen Raspberries, cooled to room temperature

Directions:

1. Place all the ingredients into a blender and pulse/beat until smooth.
2. Pour into glasses and serve.

Healthy Blueberry Pancakes

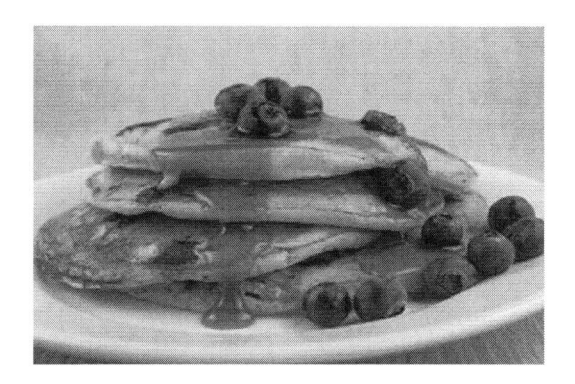

Cooking Minutes: *35 minutes*

Preparation Time: *10 minutes*

Calorie per Serving: *108 Calories*

Makes 10 Pancakes

Ingredients:

200 grams (7 ounces) Self-Rising Flour

Knob of Low-Fat Butter, melted

150 grams (5.3 ounces) Blueberries

1 teaspoon Flora Cooking Spray

Golden or Maple Syrup

1 teaspoon Baking Powder

Pinch of Salt

1 Egg

300 ml (1¼ cups) Low-Fat Milk

Directions:

1. In a large bowl, mix together the self-rising flour, a teaspoon baking powder and a pinch of salt. Beat the egg with the milk, make a well in the center of the dry ingredients and whisk in the milk to make a thick batter of smooth texture. Whisk in the melted butter, and slowly mix in half of the blueberries.
2. Heat a teaspoon of oil or small knob of butter/ Flora Cooking Spray in a large non-stick frying pan.
3. Drop a large tablespoonful of the batter per pancake into the pan to make pancakes about 7 to 7.5cm across. Make three or four pancakes each time. Allow to cook for approximately 3 minutes on medium heat until small bubbles appear on the surface of the pancakes, then turn over or flip and allow cook another 3 minutes or until golden in color.
4. Cover with kitchen paper to keep warm while you use up the rest of the batter.
5. Serve with golden syrup and the rest of the blueberries.

Tasty Baked Veggies

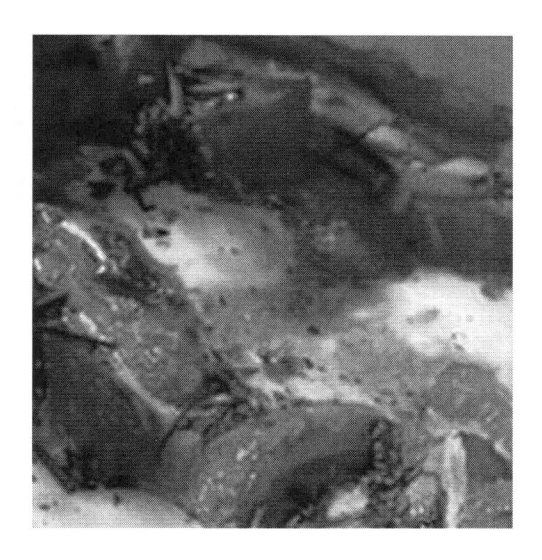

***Cooking Minutes:** 30 minutes*

***Preparation Time:** 15 minutes*

***Calorie per serving:** 127 Calories*

Makes 2 Servings

Ingredients:

1 tablespoon Olive Oil

100 grams (3.5 ounces) Spinach

2 Medium Eggs

2 Large Field Mushrooms

4 Small-Medium Tomatoes, halved

½ Garlic Clove, thinly sliced

Salt and pepper to taste

Directions:

1. Preheat oven to 200 degrees Celsius.
2. Place the large field mushrooms and halved tomatoes into 4 ovenproof/oven-safe dishes.
3. Divide thinly sliced garlic cloves evenly among the 4 dishes and sprinkle over with the olive oil and some seasoning.
4. Place dishes in the oven and bake for 10 minutes.
5. Place the spinach into a large strainer/colander, then pour over a kettle of boiling water to wilt it. Squeeze to remove excess water and then add the spinach to the dishes.
6. Create a tiny gap between the vegetables and crack an egg into each dish.
7. Return the dish to the oven and cook for a further 8 to 10 minutes or until the egg is cooked to your preference.

Guilt-Free Egg Sandwich

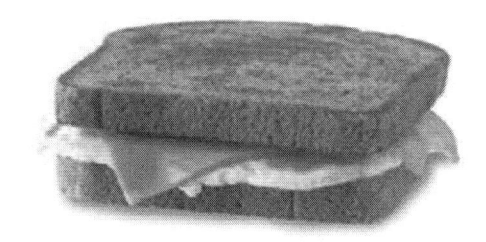

Cooking Minutes: *1 minutes*

Preparation Time: *5 minutes*

Calorie per Serving: *145 Calories*

Makes 1 Sandwich

Ingredients:

2 Egg Whites (about ¼ cup)

2 slices 100% Whole Wheat Bread (not exceeding 45 calories)

1 slice Fat-Free Cheddar Cheese

Salt and pepper to taste

Directions:

1. Pop the bread in the toaster.
2. Measure ¼ cup egg whites into bowl (you may buy the container of egg whites).
3. Place in the microwave for about 50 seconds or until you have it the way you prefer Top w/ salt and pepper.
4. Sprinkle your cooked egg whites with salt and pepper.
5. Put your sandwich together with cheese and egg when toast is done.

Peachy Citrus Smoothie

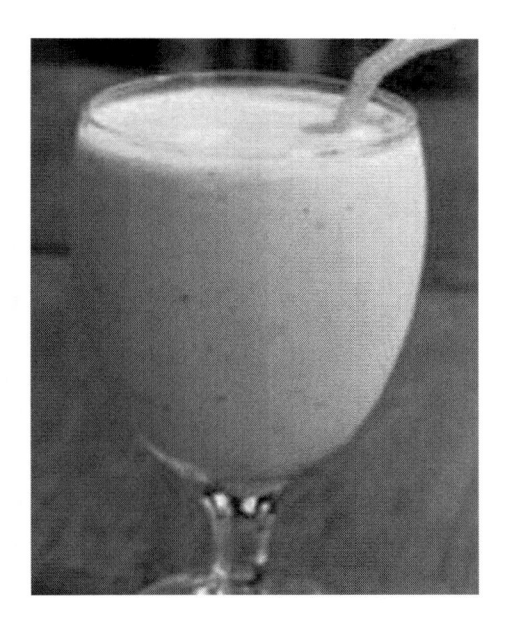

Calorie per Serving: *143 Calories*

Makes 2 Servings

Ingredients:

1½ cup (12 ounces / 355 ml) Almond Milk

1 Peach, peeled and chopped

1 Orange, peeled and chopped, seeds removed

1 Lemon, peeled and chopped, seeds removed

4 Spinach Leaves

2 Carrots, peeled and chopped (or grated)

Directions:

Blend all ingredients together.

Cheddar & Beans Omelet

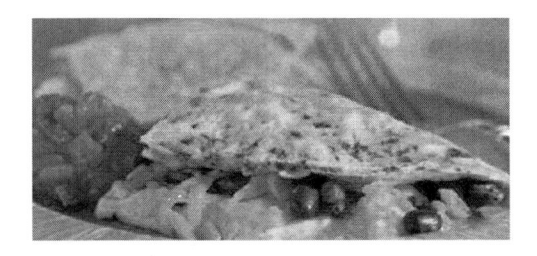

Cooking Minutes: *5 to 7 minutes*

Preparation Time: *10 minutes*

Calorie per Serving: *181 Calories*

Makes 2 Servings

Ingredients:

2 tablespoons Fresh Cilantro, chopped

½ cup (4 ounces / 113g) Canned Black Beans, rinsed thoroughly and drained of water

¼ cup (59 grams) Green Onions, chopped

¼ cup (59 grams) shredded Reduced-Fat Cheddar Cheese

¼ cup (59 grams) Bottled Salsa

¼ teaspoon Salt

4 large Egg Whites

1 large Egg

Flora cooking spray

Directions:

1. Combine cilantro, salt, egg whites and whole egg in a medium sized bowl while whisking.

2. In a separate bowl, add black beans, green onions, shredded cheese, bottled salsa and combine in a medium bowl.

3. Heat a medium nonstick skillet coated with cooking spray over medium heat. Pour egg mixture into skillet and allow egg mixture set slightly.

4. Tilt pan and carefully lift edges of omelet with a spatula/egg lifter while allowing uncooked portion to flow underneath the part that is cooked. Allow to cook for approximately 3 minutes.

5. Flip omelet. Spoon in bean mixture onto half of the omelet. Carefully loosen omelet with a spatula/egg lifter and fold in half to make omelet shape.

6. Cook for another 1 minute or until cheese is melted. Place omelet on a plate and share in half.

Raspberry Banana Smoothie

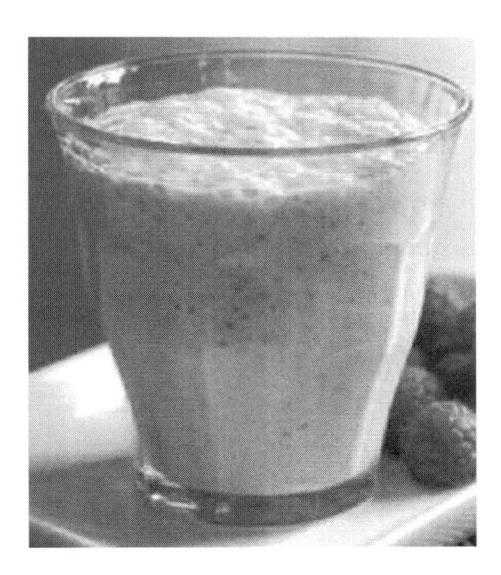

Preparation Time: *10 minutes*

Calorie per Serving: *185 Calories*

Makes 1 Serving

Ingredients:

100 milliliter (1/2 cup) Almond Milk

6 Raspberries (frozen or fresh)

1 small Ripe Banana

Directions:

1. Place almond milk in a jug and then add the rest of the ingredients.
2. Blend well in a blender until smooth and serve.

FAST DIET LUNCH & DINNERS UNDER 250 CALORIES

Holiday Zesty Honey Gammon

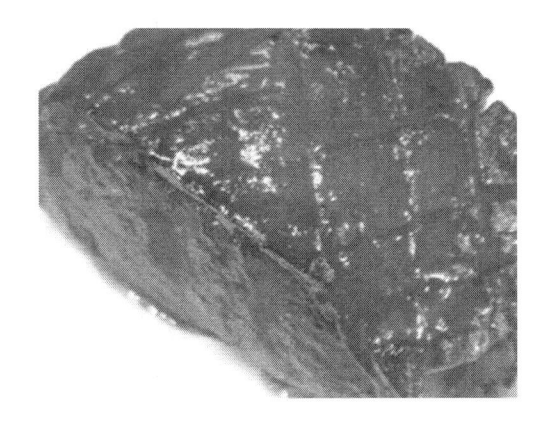

Cooking Time: 1 hour 45 minutes

Preparation Time: 3 hours 15 minutes

Calorie per Serving: 234 Calories

Makes 7 Servings *(divide as equally as possible)*

Ingredients:

0.9 kg /2 pounds Gammon Joint (cured cut from the hind leg of the pig or ham shank/hock)

1 Onion

10 Clove garlic

1 Bay Leaf

5 Peppercorns

Glaze:

20 grams / ¾ ounce / 1 tablespoon Brown Sugar (soft)

Grated rind and juice of 1/2 of a large Orange

1 tablespoon Runny Honey

1 tablespoon Wholegrain Mustard

Directions:

1. Place the gammon joint in a bowl of cold water to soak approximately 3 hours. After 3 hours, drain all liquid and put the soaked gammon in a saucepan.

2. Stud the whole onion with 2 garlic cloves and add to the saucepan along with the bay leaf and 5 peppercorns. Cover the saucepan ingredients with water, bring to boil point then use a lid to cover it. Allow to simmer for about an hour.

3. Preheat your oven to 200º Celsius or 400º Fahrenheit/gas mark
4. Prepare a roasting tin. Remove liquid from the gammon by draining and also remove any fat trimmings from the skin or elsewhere. Make diamond cuts on the gammon and pierce with the leftover cloves then place in the prepared roasting tin.
5. Combine the glaze ingredients use a spoon to pour it over the gammon. Place in the oven and bake for approximately 45 minutes while basting occasionally for 3-4 times during the cooking time. Serve as desired.

Italian Seasoned Red Potato

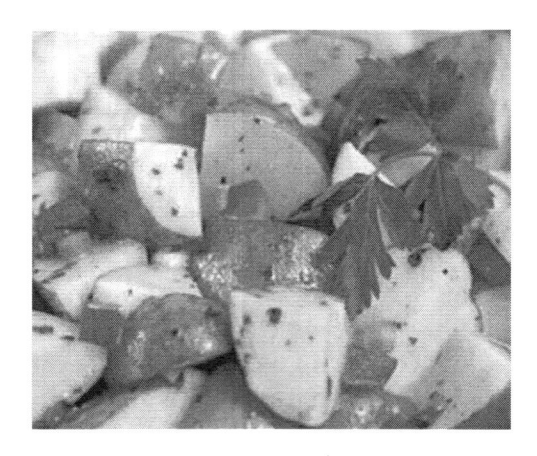

Cooking Minutes: *10 minutes*

Preparation Time: *10 minutes*

Calorie per Serving: *132 Calories*

Makes 2 Servings(1/2 cup per serving)

Ingredients:

½ pound (226 grams) (about 2-3 potatoes) Red Potatoes, diced into chunk-style

2-3 tablespoons (30 - 45 ml) Italian Salad Dressing (low calorie)

2 teaspoons (10 grams) Spicy Brown Mustard

1/3 tablespoon (5 grams) fresh Parsley, chopped

Pinch Garlic Salt or to taste

Small pinch Ground Black Pepper

2 tablespoons (30 grams) chopped Red Bell Pepper

2 tablespoons (30 grams) chopped Green Bell Pepper

2 tablespoons (30 grams) chopped Green Onions

Directions:

1. In a saucepan, cook potatoes in boiling water for about 10 minutes, until tender (do not overcook). Drain well and let cool.
2. In a small bowl, combine salad dressing, mustard, parsley, garlic salt and black pepper, then pour this over cooked potatoes and stir.
3. Gently stir in bell peppers and onions. Cover and chill until serving.

Mustard Turkey Cottage

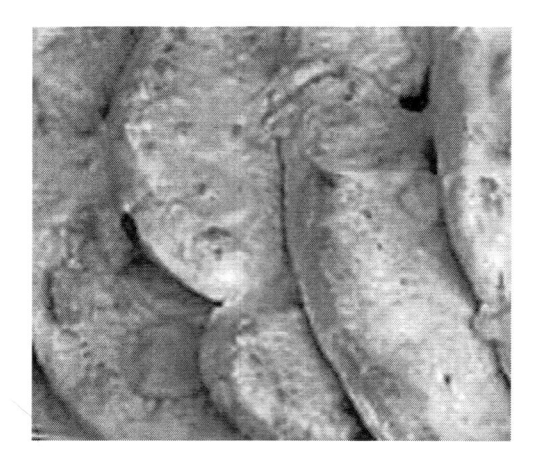

Cooking Minutes: *20 minutes*

Preparation Time: *10 minutes*

Calorie per Serving: *230 Calories*

Makes 2 Servings

Ingredients:

300 grams (10.5 ounces) Turkey Fillets

4 teaspoons (20 ml) Mustard

2 teaspoons (7 grams) Nonfat Cottage Cheese

1 tablespoon (15 ml) Olive Oil

½ tablespoon (7.5 ml) Water (add a little more if needed)

Salt to taste

Pepper to taste

Directions:

1. Grease a skillet with a tablespoon of olive oil and bring to heat over medium heat. Season the turkey fillet and fry on both sides in the heated skillet until browned. Place the browned turkey fillet aside.
2. In a bowl, thoroughly whisk mustard with cheese and 1/2 tablespoon of water until you get a evenly creamy mixture.
3. Brush each side of the browned fillet with the mustard sauce and return it to the skillet for a couple of minutes or less. Serve as warm as possible.

Easy Chili Scallops

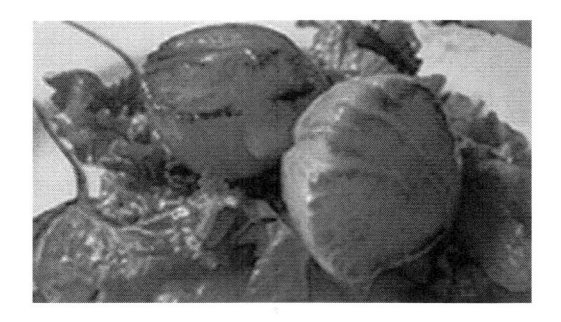

Cooking Minutes: *5 minutes*

Preparation Time: *15 minutes*

Calorie per Serving: *146 Calories*

Makes 2 Servings (3 scallops per serving)

Ingredients:

6 scallops

7.5 grams / ¼ ounce Butter, softened

½ tablespoon Olive Oil

½ of a Green Chili, finely chopped

Grated rind and juice ½ Lime

Salt

Freshly Ground Black Pepper

Rocket or Lettuce Leaves for serving

Directions:

1. Clean the scallops thoroughly and remove any unwanted portion from the scallops.

2. Whisk together the chili, butter, oil, lime rind and lime juice in a bowl and ensure that it is properly combined.

3. Bring a non-stick skillet to heat and stir in the butter mixture and heat until it reaches to boiling point. Next add in the scallops and cook on each side for approximately a minute.

4. Take the scallop from the skillet and garnish with rocket or lettuce leaves. Sprinkle a little of the scallop juices/sauce from the skillet over the meal.

Porky Chestnut Stew

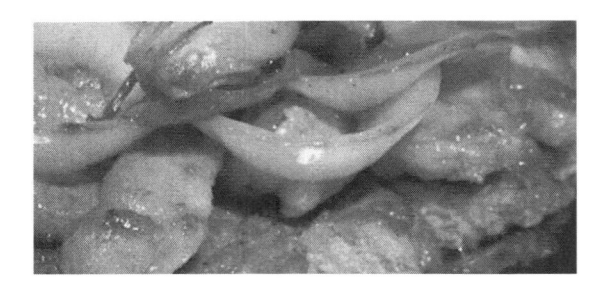

Cooking Minutes: *10 minutes*

Preparation Time: *10 minutes*

Calorie per Serving: *248 Calories*

Makes 2 Servings

Ingredients:

150 grams / 5 ½ ounce Pork Tenderloin, cut into desired slices

1 Red Pepper, sliced

1 Green Pepper, sliced

3 Bok Choi (150 grams / 5 1/2 ounces), roughly chopped

1 teaspoon Sunflower Oil

1 clove Garlic, crushed

1 teaspoon Fresh Ginger, finely chopped

3 Spring Onions, sliced

110 grams canned Water Chestnuts, drained properly and cut in halves

Sauce Ingredients:

1 tablespoon Soft Light-brown Sugar

1 tablespoon White Wine Vinegar

100 ml / 3 ½ ounces Chicken Stock

1 teaspoon Tomato Puree

1 teaspoon Corn flour

Directions:

1. Add in crushed garlic, chopped ginger and pork in a non-stick skillet and allow to cook for 4 minutes until the pork begins to achieve a brown color.
2. Next, add in the water chestnuts, sprig onions, peppers and bok choi. Allow to cook for another 3 or 4 minutes so that the vegetables are cooked.
3. Combine all the sauce ingredients and add to the content in the skillet. Allow all this to simmer for about 1-2 minutes so that the sauce becomes thickened.

Beefy Barbeque Lettuce Wraps

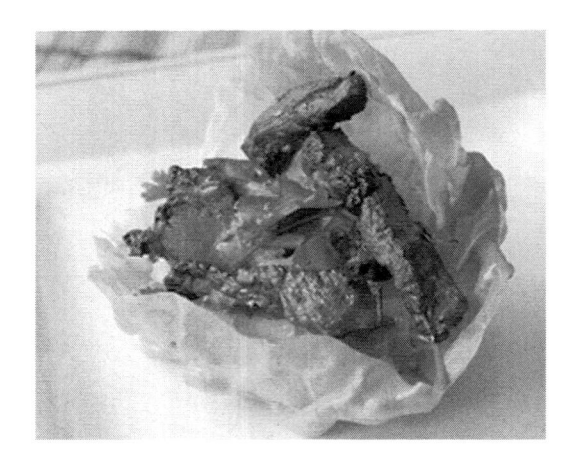

Cooking Minutes: *2 minutes*

Preparation Time: *20 minutes*

Calorie per Serving: *173 Calories*

Makes 2 Servings (2 lettuce wraps per serving)

Ingredients:

100 grams / 3.5 ounces Lean Sirloin Steak, cut into thin slices to get a few slices

1 teaspoon Sesame Oil

1/8 teaspoon Black Pepper (freshly ground)

1 Spring Onions, finely sliced

½ tablespoon Soy Sauce

¼ teaspoon Chili Flakes

¼ teaspoon Sugar

¼ tablespoon Sesame Seeds (toasted)

½ Clove Garlic, finely sliced

4 Lettuce Leaves

Directions:

1. Put the sirloin steak into a bowl and combine with ½ teaspoon sesame oil and half of the ground black pepper. Place aside for about 15 minutes.
2. Properly combine all the other ingredients in a small bowl.
3. Heat a skillet and add the sirloin steak and cook for about 2 minutes or according to your preference.
4. For serving, put slices of sirloin steak on a lettuce leaf and add a small amount of the spring onion combination, fold/wrap lettuce leaf to hold its content and enjoy. Cooked rice is a great accompaniment for this dish.

Herb Baked Cod

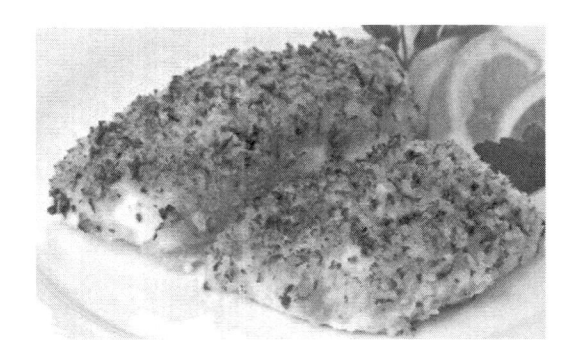

Cooking Minutes: 10-12 minutes

Preparation Time: 10 minutes

Calorie per Serving: 154 Calories

Makes 2 Servings(1 cod fillet per serving)

Ingredients:

1 tablespoon Creamed Horseradish

Granary Breadcrumbs made from 1 slice Granary Bread

1 tablespoon Fresh Parsley, chopped

2 x 125 grams / 4½ ounces chunky Cod Fillet

Salt to taste

Freshly Ground Black Pepper to taste

Directions:

1. Preheat your oven to 200° Celsius or 400° Fahrenheit/gas mark 6. Prepare a baking sheet.
2. Combine well the horseradish, Granary breadcrumbs and fresh parsley, mix thoroughly and use it to coat the cod fillets.
3. Put on the prepared baking sheet and bake for 11 minutes or until the cod fillet is properly cooked.
4. Serve as desired with low calorie rice or veggies.

Sweet 'n' Spicy Salmon

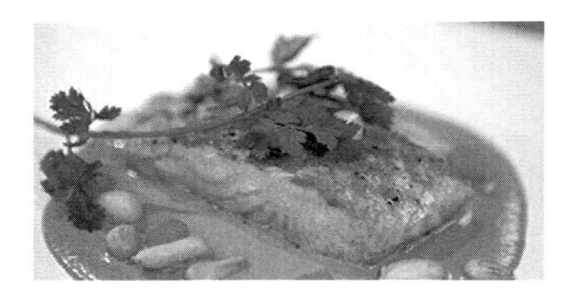

Cooking Minutes: *3-4 minutes*

Preparation Time: *10 minutes*

Calorie per Serving: *246 Calories*

Makes 2 Servings (1 Salmon Fillet per serving)

Ingredients:

2 pieces Salmon Fillet (42 grams (1½ ounce) each

2/3 tablespoons Soy Sauce

2/3 teaspoons Sesame Oil

Small pinch Chili flakes

1/3 teaspoon Fresh Ginger, grated

2/3 teaspoons Runny Honey

1/3 tablespoon fresh chopped Coriander

1 Spring Onions, shredded

Directions:

1. Place the following ingredients in a bowl (non-metallic): soy sauce, sesame oil, pinch chili flakes, fresh ginger, and honey. Mix thoroughly.
2. Add the 2 salmon fillets, evenly coat in the soy sauce marinade mixture and place aside.
3. In a skillet, allow to cook for 3½ minutes on medium heat on each side while brushing at intervals with any leftover soy sauce marinade mixture.
4. Top with the coriander and spring onions, garnish as desired and serve.

Spicy Turkey Cooked Vegetables

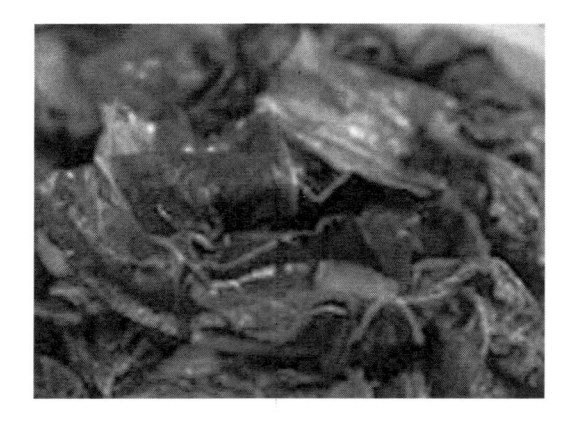

Cooking Minutes: *30 minutes*

Preparation Time: *10 minutes*

Calorie per Serving: *69 Calories*

**Makes 3 Servings(1 cup per serving)*

Ingredients:

1½ cups (360 ml) Water

2 ounces (56 grams) of Smoked Turkey Breast, without skin

1/8 cup (30 grams) chopped Onion

½ tablespoon (7.5 grams) minced Jalapeno Pepper (optional)

1 Clove Garlic, minced

1/8 teaspoon Cayenne Pepper

1/8 teaspoon Ground Cloves

¼ teaspoon Thyme

½ of a Green Onion, chopped

½ teaspoon Ground Ginger

1 pound (453 grams) Cabbage or Kale or a mixture of both

Directions:

1. Put all ingredients, except leafy vegetables in a large saucepan and bring to a boil.
2. Prepare washing leafy vegetables thoroughly and removing stems. Cut the leaves into small pieces.
3. Add greens to turkey stock. Cook 20 to 30 minutes until tender. Please serve hot.

Vegan Creamed Tortilla Wraps

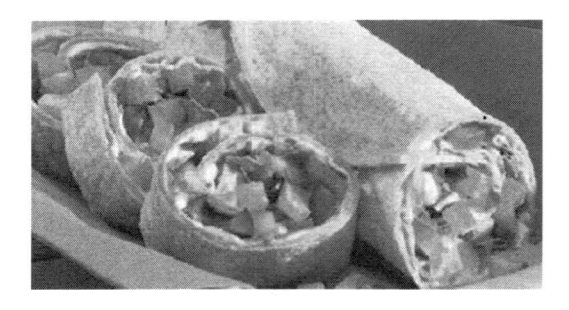

Cooking Minutes: *10 minutes*

Preparation Time: *10 minutes*

Calorie per Serving: *128 Calories*

**Makes 2 Servings*(1 tortilla roll per serving)*

Ingredients:

2 Whole Wheat Tortillas Wraps (7 inch)

4 tablespoons (1/4 cup / 60 ml) fat free Cream Cheese

1 cup (236 grams) Romaine Lettuce cut into julienne or thin strips, or chopped Fresh Spinach

½ cup (118 grams) chopped Tomato

¼ cup (59 grams) chopped Bell Pepper (red or yellow or a mixture)

¼ cup (59 grams) chopped Cucumber

1/8 cup (30 grams) canned Green Chilies, diced

1/8 cup (30 grams) Ripe Olives, drained

Directions:

1. Spread each tortilla with 2 tablespoons cream cheese. Top with equal amounts of vegetables.
2. Roll up to enclose filling while squeezing it firmly and serve.

Fish 'n' Veggie Tacos

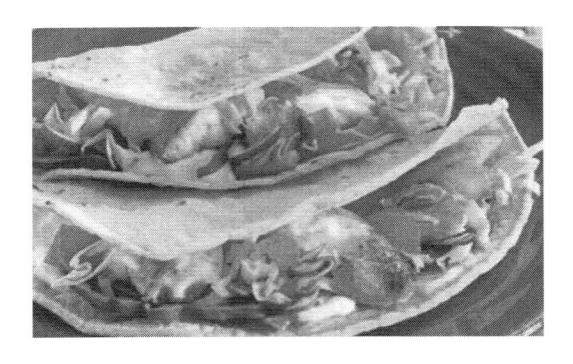

Cooking Minutes: *5 minutes*

Preparation Time: *20 minutes*

Calorie per Serving: *239 Calories*

Makes 3 Servings (2 tacos per serving)

Ingredients:

8 ounces (226 grams) White Fish Fillets, cut in 1-inch pieces

½ tablespoon (7.5 ml) Olive Oil

1 tablespoon (15 ml) Lemon Juice

¼ packet Taco Seasoning Mix (I used Mrs. Dash Taco Seasoning Mix)

6 Corn Tortillas (6-inch)

½ cup (118 grams) Purple Cabbage, cut into thin strips

½ cup (118 grams) Green Cabbage, cut into thin strips

1 cup (236 grams) chopped Tomatoes

¼ cup (60 ml) Sour Cream

Taco Sauce to taste

Green Lemon Wedges for serving (optional)

Directions:

1. In a bowl, combine the fish, olive oil, lemon juice and taco seasoning mix then place in a saucepan. Cook, stirring constantly over medium -high heat for 4 to 5 minutes, or until fish flesh is flakes easily with a fork.
2. Fill tortillas with fish mixture. Top with cabbage, tomato, sour cream and taco sauce. Serve tacos with lemon slices, if desired.

Squash Zucchini Split

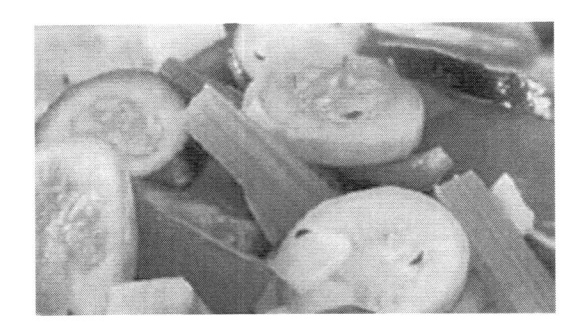

Cooking Minutes: *10 minutes*

Preparation Time: *10 minutes*

Calorie per Serving: *30 Calories*

Makes 2 Servings(1/2 cup per serving)

Ingredients:

1 tablespoon (15 ml) Water

½ cup (118 grams) Zucchini cut into thin slices

½ + 1/8 cups (147 grams) Yellow Squash cut into thin slices

¼ cup (59 grams) Green Pepper, cut into 2-inch strips

1/8 cup (30 grams) Celery cut into strips 2-inches

1/8 cup (30 grams) chopped Onion

¼ teaspoon (1.25 grams) Caraway Seeds

A small pinch Garlic Powder

½ of a medium Tomato cut into 4 wedges

Directions:

1. Heat water in a saucepan. Add zucchini, squash, pepper, celery and onion.
2. Cover with lid and allow to cook over medium heat until the squash, zucchini, pepper, celery and onion are fairly tender, approximately 4 minutes.
3. Sprinkle the seasonings over the vegetables.
4. Finally, add the tomato wedges. Cover again and let simmer until tomato is warm, about 2 minutes.
5. Serve warm.

Turkey Zucchini Bolognese

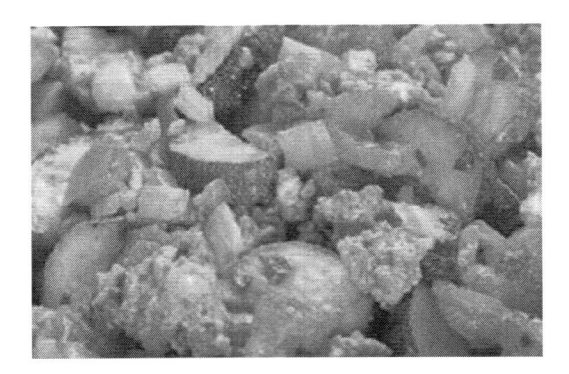

Cooking Minutes: *25 minutes*

Preparation Time: *5 minutes*

Calorie per Serving: *181 Calories*

**Makes 2 Servings(1 cup per serving)*

Ingredients:

Flora Cooking Spray

6 ounces (170 grams) of Ground Turkey Meat

½ of a medium Onion, peeled and diced

1½ medium Tomatoes, chopped

1½ tablespoons (22.5 ml) Tomato Paste

¼ teaspoon Salt

1/8 teaspoon Ground Black Pepper

1 medium Zucchini, sliced

½ teaspoon (2.5 grams) of each the following seasonings:

Dried Basil

Dried Oregano

Garlic Powder

Directions:

1. Spray a skillet with cooking spray.
2. Brown turkey and onion over medium heat until meat is fully cooked and the onion tender, for about 10 minutes.
3. Add tomatoes, tomato paste and all other seasonings. Allow to cook over medium heat for 10 minutes.
4. Add zucchini and cook 5 minutes more.
5. Serve warm.

Veggie Chicken Mix

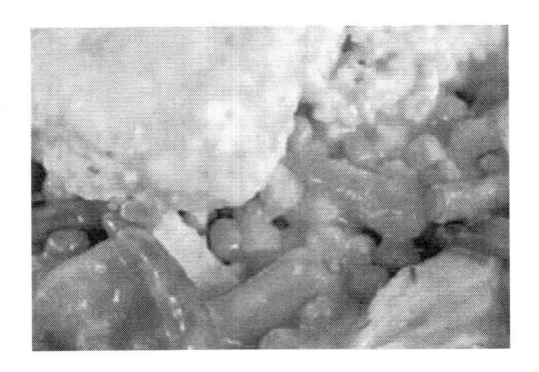

Cooking Minutes: *25 minutes*

Preparation Time: *10 minutes*

Calorie per Serving: *226 Calories*

**Makes 2 Servings(1¼ cup per serving)*

Ingredients:

¾ cup (177 ml) low sodium Chicken Broth

2 tablespoons (30 ml) Water

1/3 of a Medium Onion, peeled and chopped

1½ cups (354 grams) of frozen Mixed Vegetables

2/3 cup (158 grams) Cooked Chicken Breasts, chopped

1/3 teaspoon (a small pinch) Dried Thyme

1/2 cup (75 grams) Baking Mix

1-2 tablespoons (15 – 30 ml) Low-fat Milk

1 Egg White

Directions:

1. In a saucepan, combine chicken broth, water, onion, mixed vegetables, chicken and thyme.
2. Cover and bring to a boil over medium -high then reduce heat and let simmer for 15 minutes.
3. Place baking mix in a small bowl. Put 2 teaspoons of the baking mix diluted with 4 teaspoons of water in the saucepan and mix it well to thicken the stew. Add milk and egg whites to remaining baking mix, and whisk with a fork. Add more liquid if necessary to make dough that is not dry.
4. Add heaping tablespoons of the dough mixture in the hot stew. Simmer, without lid for 5 minutes.
5. Cover and continue cooking for another 5 minutes. Serve warm.

Sweet Turkey Pepper Bowl

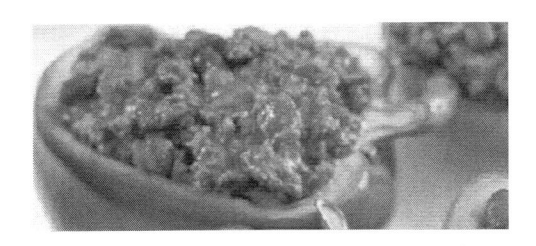

Cooking Minutes: 25 minutes

Preparation Time: 10 minutes

Calorie per Serving: 209 Calories

Makes 2 Servings (1/2 stuffed pepper per serving)

Ingredients:

¼ pound (113 grams) of lean Ground Turkey Meat

1/3 of a Large Onion, peeled and chopped

1/3 of a medium Green Pepper, seeds removed and chopped

5 ounces (141 grams) canned dice Tomatoes (unsalted)

1/3 cup (78 ml) low-sodium Black Beans, drained and rinsed

1/8 cup + 1 tablespoon (45 ml) Barbecue Sauce (homemade is best)

Small pinch Garlic Powder

1 teaspoon (6 ml) Liquid Smoke

1 Sweet Peppers (any color)

Flora Cooking Spray

Directions:

1. Spray cooking spray in a heated saucepan and brown the ground turkey in a pan over medium to medium-high heat until no longer pink, discard the excess fat/oil.
2. Add onion and cook for 5 minutes, until tender.
3. Add remaining ingredients except whole pepper and cook over medium heat for 10 minutes.
4. Meanwhile, cut the whole sweet pepper in half lengthwise and remove the seeds. Put the halved pepper in a microwave-safe dish with a small amount of water. Cover and cook for about 5 minutes in the microwave at high power until pepper is tender -crisp.
5. Remove the pepper from the dish and place on a serving platter. With a spoon, fill the peppers with the ground turkey mixture and serve.

Deluxe Thai Salad

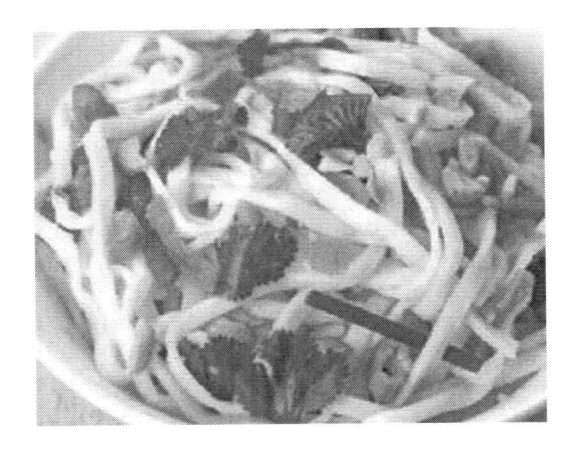

Cooking Minutes: *15 minutes*

Preparation Time: *15 minutes*

Calorie per Serving: *192 Calories*

Makes 2 Servings

Ingredients:

2 tablespoons Thai Vegetarian Paste Sauce/Thai Fish Sauce

1 Red Chili, finely shredded

1 large Carrot, finely shredded or grated

50 gram (1.8 ounces) bundles, Rice Vermicelli Noodles (soaked/prepared according to the package instructions)

½ of a Small Bunch Mint/Coriander, chopped

½ handful Peanuts, toasted and chopped (optional – Roasted Sesame Seed can also be used)

1 small Lime (1-2 teaspoon), juiced

½ tablespoon Stevia (Raw Agave can also be used)

1 Shallot, finely sliced

Directions:

1. In a large bowl, put the vegetarian paste/fish sauce, lime juice, stevia/raw agave, shallots and chilies and leave to sit for 5 minutes.
2. Add the carrots, drained noodles and mint/coriander and toss everything together. Top with the peanuts/sesame seed if you desired.
3. Serve

Avocado Tortilla Chowder

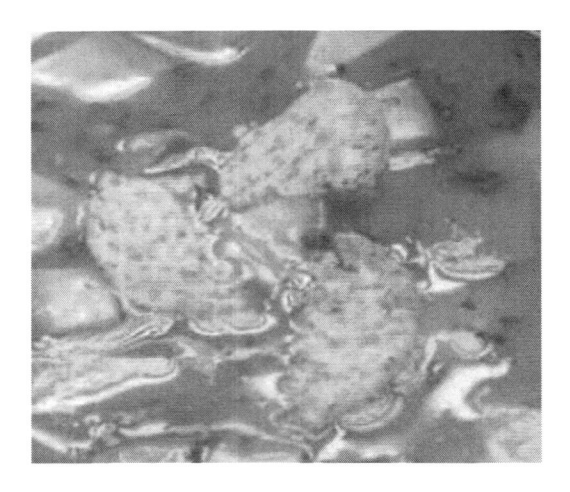

Cooking Minutes: *15 minutes*

Preparation Time: *15 minutes*

Calorie per Serving: *134 Calories*

Makes 2 Servings *(1 cup per serving)*

Ingredients:

10.5 ounces (310 ml) reduced sodium Chicken Broth

2¾ ounces (81 ml) of canned low sodium Tomato Condensed Soup

1/8 bunch Cilantro, only leaves

1 Clove Garlic, finely chopped

1/8 teaspoon (small dash) Ground Black Pepper

¼ of a ripe Avocado, peeled and chopped

2 Corn Tortilla Chips broken in pieces

<u>Directions:</u>

1. In a skillet over high heat , combine chicken broth, the tomato soup , cilantro , garlic and black pepper .
2. Bring to a boil , reduce heat and let simmer for 10 minutes.
3. Let cool slightly and then in small portions liquefy in a blender.
4. Put back into the pan, add the avocado and heat it well .
5. With a ladle , serve it in soup bowls and garnish with bits of tortilla chips before serving.

Spicy Vegetable Bowl

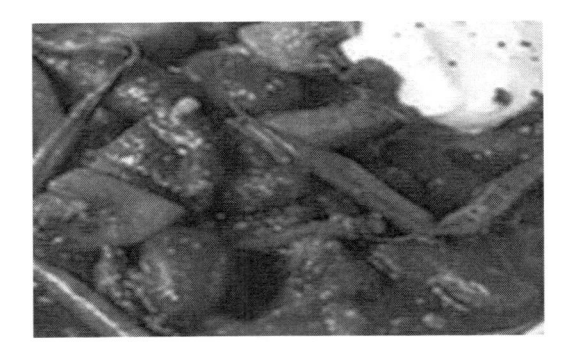

Cooking Minutes: *20 minutes*

Preparation Time: *10 minutes*

Calorie per Serving: *133 Calories*

Makes 3 Servings

Ingredients:

250 grams (8.8 ounces) Chestnut Mushrooms, cut into quarter pieces

400 grams (14.1 ounces) tin of Chopped Tomatoes

400 grams (14.1 ounces) tin of Kidney Beans

150 grams (5.3 ounces) Green Beans, cut into lengths

2 Garlic Cloves, crushed

2 Red Chilies, finely chopped

1 tablespoon Extra Virgin Olive Oil

2 teaspoon Ground Cumin

A drop (or more) Half-Fat Crème Fraîche/Light Sour Cream, to serve

Salt to taste

Directions:

1. Fry the garlic and chili in 1 tablespoon olive oil for approximately 2 minutes. Add in the ground cumin and chestnut mushrooms and cook for about 3 minutes.
2. Add the tomatoes, kidney beans and 200ml / ¾ cup water or water drained from kidney beans, stir with a spoon and allow to simmer for 10 minutes.
3. Add the green beans and cook for another 5 minutes until the sauce is thickened and vegetable is cooked according to your liking.
4. Serve in bowls with a drop of crème fraîche/light sour cream. You may serve low calorie toasted whole wheat bread/crusty bread.

Asian Style Chicken Salad

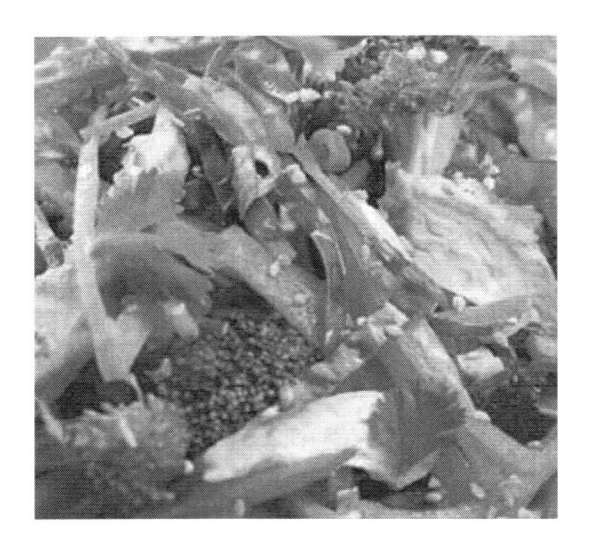

Cooking Minutes: *None*

Preparation Time: *20 minutes*

Calorie per Serving: *184 Calories*

Makes 2 Servings *(1 cup per serving)*

Ingredients:

1 cooked Chicken Breast, boneless, skinless and shredded (cold temperature)

1 Green Onion, chopped

¾ cup (177 grams) small clusters Broccoli

1 medium Carrots, peeled and cut into strips

½ of a Red Pepper, cut into strips

1 cup (236 grams) Cabbage cut in thin strips

¼ cup (59 grams) fat free Asian Sesame Salad dressing

1/8 cup (30 ml) freshly squeezed Orange Juice

1/8 cup (30 grams) Fresh Cilantro, chopped

Directions:

1. Place the chicken breast strips in a medium bowl with onion, broccoli, carrot, bell pepper and cabbage.
2. In a small bowl, mix the salad dressing with the squeezed orange juice then pour it into the salad and mix well. Stir in the cilantro and serve.

Creamy Orange Carrot Soup

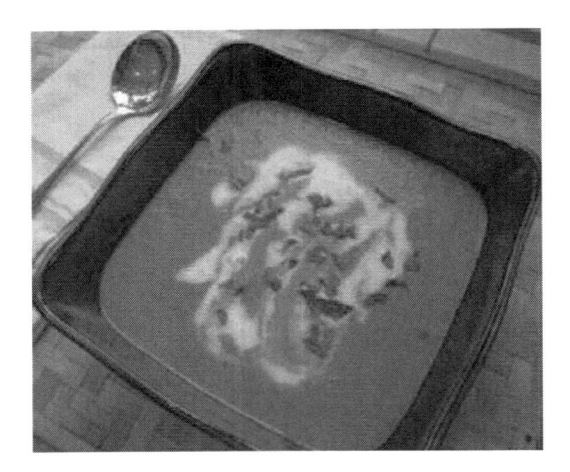

Cooking Minutes: *45 minutes*

Preparation Time: *45 minutes to 1 hour*

Calorie per Servings: *120 Calories*

Makes 4 Servings

Ingredients:

Small knob of Low-Fat Butter (about 1/8 stick)

700 grams (1.5 pounds) Carrots, peeled and thinly sliced

1 large Onion, thinly sliced

1 large Garlic Clove, crushed

1 liter(4¼ cups)Light Vegetable Stock

125 ml (1/2 cup) freshly Squeezed Orange Juice

2 tablespoons finely Chopped Fresh Mint (if preferred)

Double cream, for drizzling (if preferred)

Directions:

1. In a medium saucepan, spray about 2 teaspoons of Flora Cooking Spray gently then add the thinly sliced carrots, onion and crushed garlic clove. Put a lid or cover on the saucepan and leave on a low heat for about 12 minutes, stirring occasionally, until the vegetables have softened but not colored.
2. Pour in the stock and sprinkle in a little salt. Bring to boiling point and allow to simmer, partly covered, for about 25 minutes or until the vegetables are properly cooked. Remove from the heat and allow to cool for a few minutes.
3. Strain the vegetables through a sieve that is placed over a bowl. Keep the liquid. Place the vegetables in a food processor or blender. Process until smooth while adding enough of the strained liquid to make the mixture turn easily in the machine.
4. Set the sieve over the cleaned pan and push the puréed vegetables through (this step is optional but gives the soup a texture that is smooth). Stir in the liquid and combine thoroughly.
5. Pour in the orange juice and mint and bring back heat to the soup. Mix and taste in order to see if more salt may be needed, then pour into warmed bowls. If you would like to add the double cream, you can sprinkle a little over the top.

Lemon Smoked Salmon

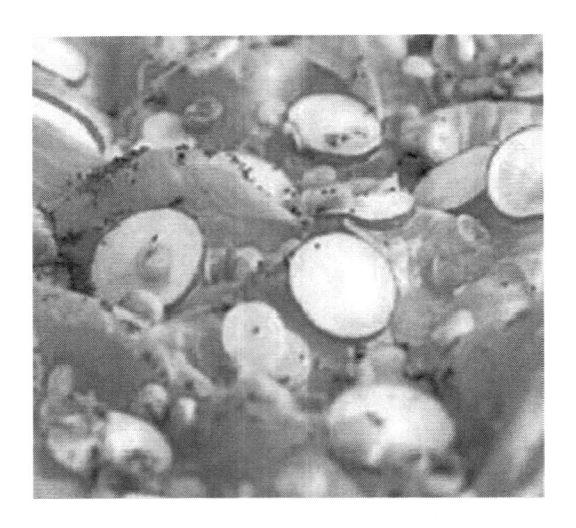

Preparation Time: *15 minutes*

Calorie per Servings: *99 Calories*

Makes 5 servings

Ingredients:

1 tablespoon Poppy Seed, lightly toasted

½ teaspoon Sesame Oil

300 grams (10.5 ounces) Smoked Salmon

85 grams (3 ounces) Radishes, trimmed and finely sliced

2 spring Onions, finely sliced

1 Orange, freshly juice

1 teaspoon Red Wine Vinegar

2 teaspoon Olive Oil

Black Pepper to taste

Salt to taste (optional)

Directions:

1. In a bowl, whisk together the poppy seeds, orange juice, vinegar and oils with some black pepper and a pinch of salt - be sparing with the salt.
2. Carefully separate the slices of salmon and then put into a mixing bowl with most of the radishes and spring onions. Sprinkle over the dressing and gently toss together lightly - using your hands is best. Let the salmon marinate for just 5-10 minutes.
3. Spread the salmon over a large plate or platter; pour over any dressing that remains in the bowl, then add the reserved radishes and spring onions on top.
4. Serve with toasted low calorie bread.

Minty Green Pea Soup

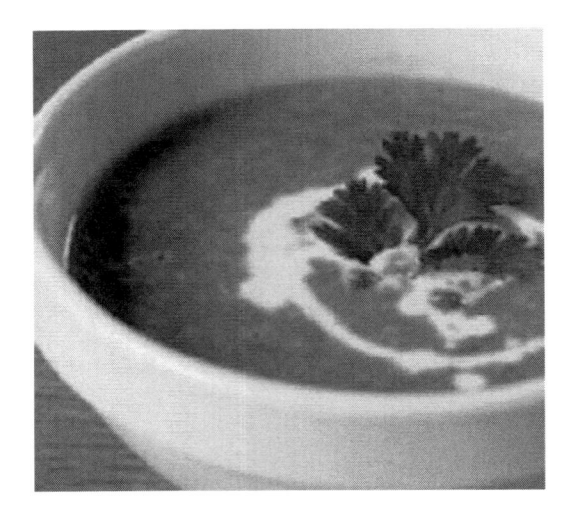

Cooking Minutes: *20 minutes*

Preparation Time: *10 minutes*

Calorie count: *108 Calories*

Makes 4 Servings

Ingredients:

900 grams (2 pounds) Young Peas in the pod (250g/9oz shelled peas)

4 tablespoon Fresh Mint, chopped

Large pinch Stevia/Raw Agave

1 teaspoon Fresh Lemon or Lime Juice

150 ml (1/2 cup + 2 tablespoons) Buttermilk or Sour Cream

1 bunch Spring Onions, trimmed and roughly chopped

1 medium Irish Potato, peeled and diced

1 Garlic Clove, crushed

850 ml (4 cups + 1 tablespoon) Vegetable or Chicken Stock

Salt to taste

Pepper to taste

Directions:

1. In a large bowl, add the spring onions, the potato, garlic and stock. Bring to boiling point, lower the heat and allow to simmer for approximately 15 minutes or until the potato is very soft.
2. For the garnish, blanch 3 tablespoon of the shelled peas in boiling water for about 3 minutes, drain, place in a bowl of cold water and place aside. Add in the remaining peas to the soup base and simmer for approximately 5 minutes - no longer, or you may lose the lovely fresh flavor of the peas.
3. Stir in the mint, stevia and lemon juice (or lime juice), allow to cool slightly, then transfer into a food processor or liquidizer and process until as smooth according to your liking. Stir in half the buttermilk or sour cream, taste and season with salt and pepper.
4. To serve the soup cold, cool quickly and then chill -

you may need to add more stock to the soup before serving as it will begin to get thicker while cooling. Serve hot by reheating the soup without boiling. This may help to prevent the buttermilk or soured cream from curdling.

5. Serve as desired, garnished with the remaining buttermilk and the drained peas.

Delicious Vegan Coleslaw

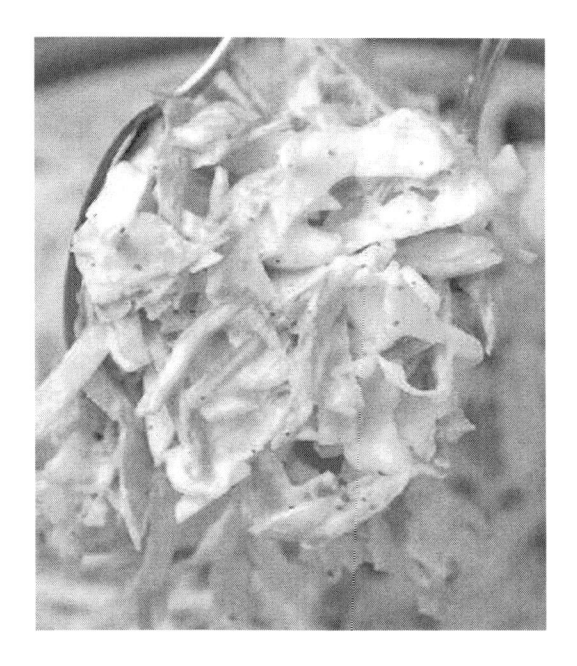

Preparation Time: *10 minutes*

Calorie count: *151 Calories*

Makes 3 Servings

Ingredients:

1½ tablespoons Low-Fat Plain Yogurt

¼ teaspoon Dijon Mustard

1½ tablespoon Reduced Fat Mayonnaise

¼ of a White Cabbage, shredded

1 medium Carrots, grated

1/8 of a medium Onion, finely chopped

¼ teaspoon White Vinegar

Directions:

1. Mix the yogurt, mustard, vinegar, olive oil and mayonnaise together in a bowl.
2. Add all of the vegetables into the bowl and stir through the dressing.

Olive Baked Potatoes

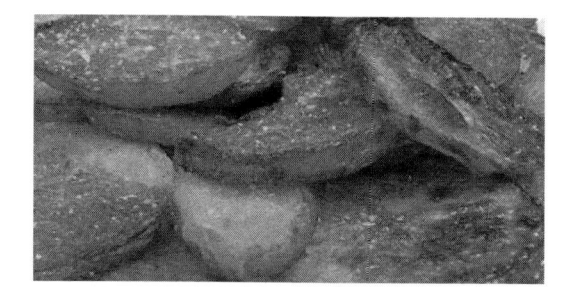

Cooking Minutes: *45 minutes*

Preparation Time: *5 minutes*

Calorie count: *187 Calories*

Makes 2 Servings

Ingredients:

2 medium Baking Potatoes

Extra Virgin Olive Oil , for drizzling

Sea Salt to taste

Directions:

1. Preheat oven to 200 degrees Celsius. Scrub the baking potatoes and pat dry. Slice lengthways into three.

2. Drizzle olive oil over a baking sheet. Arrange the potatoes on the baking sheet, drizzle with olive oil, rub all over and then generously sprinkle with sea salt.

3. Bake for 40-45 minutes (longer for extra crispiness) then turn when halfway, and bake until it becomes golden brown in colour and soft.

4. Serve as desired.

Tasty Vegetable Delight

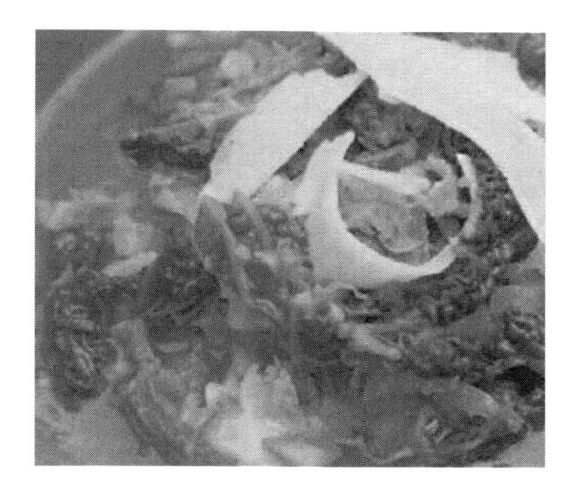

Cooking Minutes: *10 minutes*

Preparation Time: *10 minutes*

Calorie count: *169 Calories*

Makes 3 Servings

Ingredients:

1 small Savoy Cabbage, cut in quarters, cored removed and shredded

200 grams (7 ounces) canned Haricot Beans, washed and drained

150 ml (1/2 + 1/8 cups) Chicken Stock

12 grams (1/2 ounce) Flora Cooking Spray

2 rashers smoked Streaky Bacon, chopped (or strips of chicken breasts)

1 medium Carrots, peeled and chopped into small chunks

Salt and Pepper to taste

Directions:

1. In a wide saucepan, spray Flora Cooking Spray. Add the bacon/chicken and carrots and then sizzle for 3-4 minutes until the bacon/chicken starts to crisp.

2. Stir in the cabbage, cook for 2 minutes until wilted and then add the beans. Pour over the stock and then simmer for about 5 minutes until the beans are hot and the carrots are just cooked.

3. Serve as desired.

Healthy Mashed Potatoes

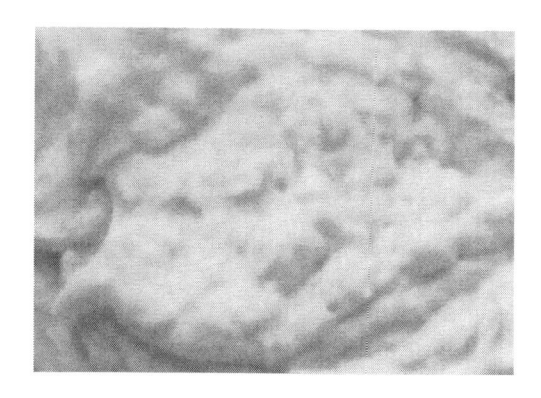

Cooking Minutes: *20 minutes*

Calorie count: *196 Calories*

Makes 2 Servings

Ingredients:

½ kg (17.5 ounces) Irish Potatoes

Splash Low-Fat Milk or Cream / Soy Cream (optional)

100 grams (3.5 ounces) Low-Fat Butter

Nutmeg (optional)

Directions:

1. Peel the potatoes and cut them into pieces evenly (approx. 3x3cm)
2. If you choose to boil the potatoes, ensure that they are properly cooked through so that they don't start getting ragged around the edges or they'll become water-logged. Afterwards drain the excess water and steam dry for a short period in the pan.
3. Once you have nice, dry, cooked potatoes add milk (or cream if you prefer) and return the pan back to the heat until the liquid becomes hot.
4. Add the butter and mash quickly (or use electric whisk) until a smooth texture is achieved. Sprinkle with a little nutmeg if you would like to.
5. Serve as desired.

Tomato and Kale Soup

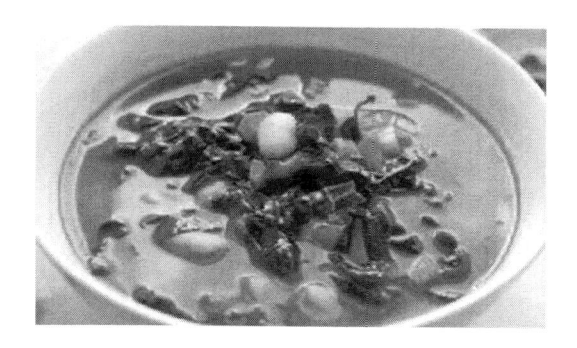

Cooking Minutes: *35 minutes*

Preparation Time: *10 minutes*

Calorie count: *145 Calories*

Makes 2 Servings

Ingredients:

1 medium Carrots, diced

200 grams (7 ounces) canned chop Tomatoes

200 grams (7 ounces) canned Borlotti Beans (or Chickpeas)

300 ml (1½ + 1/8 cups) Vegetable Stock

50 grams (1¾ ounces) Kale, washed and chopped

½ of an Onion, chopped

½ tablespoon Olive Oil

½ Garlic Clove, sliced

1 Celery Stalks, diced

Salt to taste

Directions:

1. In a deep saucepan/pot, cook the onion in olive oil until softened then add the garlic, celery and carrot and cook for a minute.
2. Add the tomatoes, beans and stock, then simmer for 20 minutes. Add the kale and simmer for another 10 minutes.
3. Serve as desired.

Lemon Beetroot Salad

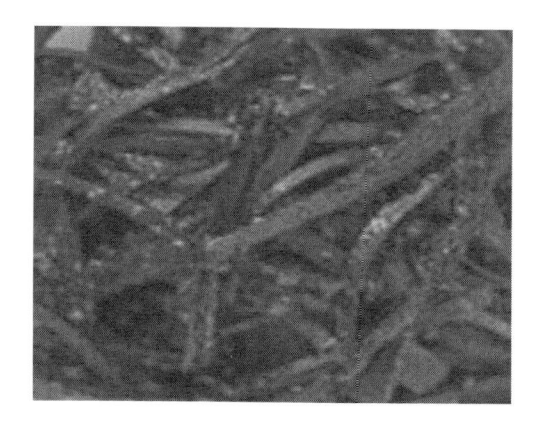

Cooking Minutes: *10 minutes*

Preparation Time: *5 minutes*

Calorie count: *44 Calories*

Makes 2 Servings

Ingredients:

1½ raw Beetroot, peeled and cut into strips

½ of a Lemon, juiced

½ tablespoon Stevia

½ tablespoon Grainy Mustard

Flora Cooking Spray

Directions:

1. In a large non-stick frying pan, spray some cooking spray and fry the beetroot for about 2 minutes.
2. Add the lemon juice and cook for another minute.
3. Drizzle in the stevia and mustard and stir to coat the beetroot.
4. Serve immediately

Spicy Prawn Soup

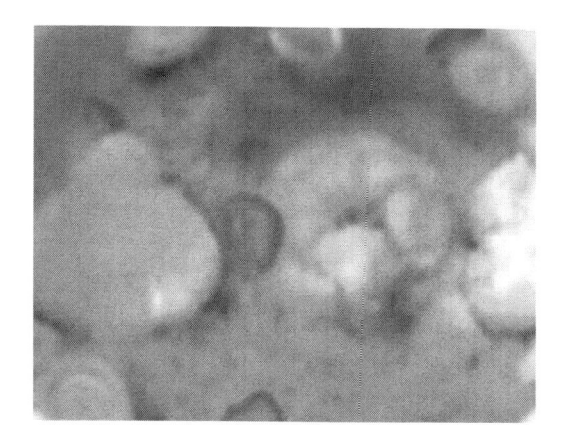

Cooking Minutes: *5 minutes*

Preparation Time: *10 minutes*

Calorie count: *93 Calories*

Makes 2 Servings

Ingredients:

½ tablespoon Stevia

½ of thumb-size piece Ginger, peeled and thinly sliced

1 small hot Red Chilies, thinly sliced

1½ Spring Onions, thinly sliced

150 grams (5¼ ounces) small Raw Peeled Prawns, from a sustainable source (Chicken Breasts can also be used)

1½ tablespoon Rice Vinegar (use White Wine Vinegar if you prefer)

250 ml (1 cup) Chicken Stock

½ tablespoon Soy Sauce

Directions:

1. In a saucepan, put the vinegar, stock, soy sauce, stevia, ginger, chilies and spring onions in a saucepan and bring to a simmer.
2. Cook for about a minute and then add the prawns to heat through.
3. Serve in small bowls or cups.

Red & Green Ham Salad

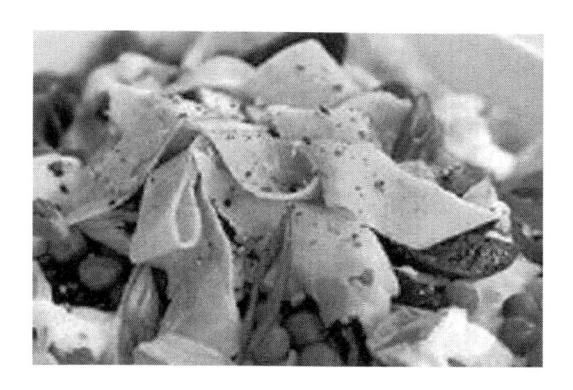

Preparation Time: *15 minutes*

Calorie count: *166 Calories*

Makes 2 Servings

Ingredients:

1 tablespoon Low-Fat Yogurt

1 teaspoon Horseradish Sauce

¼ of a iceberg Lettuce, shredded

50 grams (1.8 ounces) Wafer-Thin Sliced Ham

50 grams (1.8 ounces) Frozen Green Peas

88 grams (3.1 ounces) Beetroot, chopped into cubes

1 spring Onion, thinly sliced

Directions:

1. Pour boiling water over the peas and leave for approximately 2 minutes, afterwards, drain thoroughly.

2. In a bowl, place the peas, beetroot and spring onions into a bowl and combine thoroughly. Combine the low-fat yogurt and horseradish sauce, then add about 1 tablespoon boiling water to make a pouring sauce dressing.

3. Heap the shredded lettuce into bowls, then use a spoon to pour the beetroot mix over it. Sparingly drizzle the dressing over the salad and top with ham.

Healthy Spring Vegetable Soup

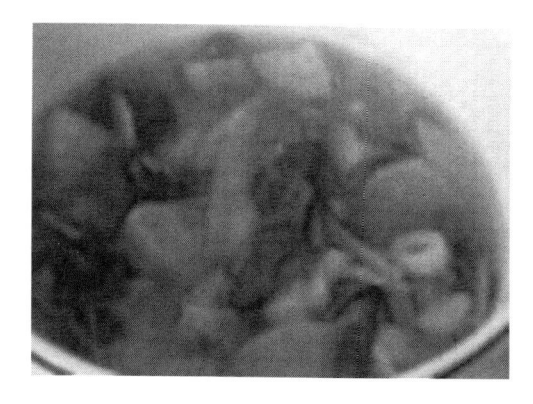

Cooking Minutes: *25 minutes*

Preparation Time: *15 minutes*

Calorie count: *80 Calories*

Makes 2 Servings

Ingredients:

¼ cup (59 grams) frozen Green Peas

¼ teaspoon Oregano

¼ teaspoon Dried Basil

¼ teaspoon Dried Thyme

1½ cups (360 ml) fat-free, low sodium Vegetable or Chicken

Broth

½ cup (118 grams) Fresh Baby Spinach

2 tablespoons Fresh Parsley, chopped

¼ teaspoon Olive Oil

½ clove garlic, minced

¼ of a small onion, diced

½ stalk Celery, chopped

1 small Leek, chopped (use the white part only)

1 small Carrots, cut in halves by length and sliced

1 small Zucchini, halved lengthwise and sliced

Kosher Salt and Pepper to taste

Directions:

1. In a pan, heat oil over medium heat. Cook garlic, carrots, celery, leeks, onions and celery until softened for about 6-7 minutes.
2. Add zucchini and sauté for another 2-3 minutes.
3. Add green peas, sprinkle dried herbs, and stir for about a minute. Add broth.
4. Bring to boil, then cover and simmer for about 10 minutes. Add in spinach and fresh parsley, give a gentle stir and allow to simmer for approximately 2 minutes.
5. Season with Kosher salt and black pepper to taste.

Special Beetroot and Bramley Soup

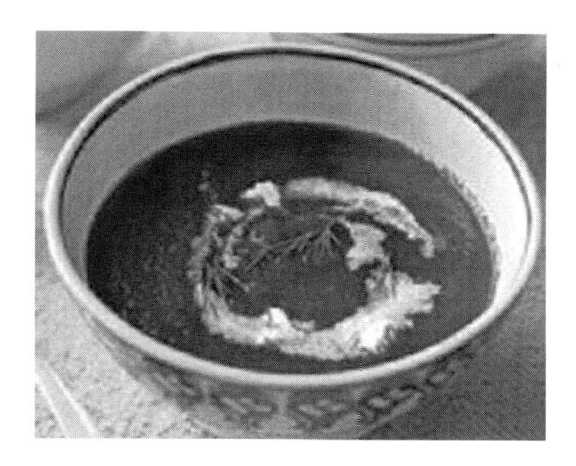

Cooking Minutes: 1½ to 1¾ hours

Preparation Time: 15-30minutes

Calorie count: 190 Calories

Makes 2 Servings

Ingredients:

¼ of small Bramley Apple

200 grams (7 ounces) Beetroot, trimmed and sliced (no peel necessary)

375 ml (1½ cups) Light Chicken Stock /Vegetable Stock, hot

Flora Cooking Spray

½ medium Onion, chopped

½ medium Carrot, chopped

½ of a Celery Stick, chopped

1½ Garlic Clove, chopped

Salt and Pepper to taste

Fresh Dill Sprigs and Low-Fat Plain Yogurt (optional)

Directions:

1. In a large, heavy-based pan in a large, spray Flora Cooking Spray on low heat. Add in the celery, carrots, garlic, onions and a little water, cover with a lid and allow it to steam/sweat for about 12-15 minutes while stirring at intervals. Cook until the onions are soft.

2. Peel, core and slice the apple and add to the pan with the beetroot. Cover and steam/sweat for a further 15 minutes.

3. Pour in the chicken/vegetable stock, season and bring to the boil. Reduce the heat and simmer, uncovered, for 1 hour or until the beetroot is tender.

4. Cool slightly, then purée with a hand blender or in a food processor in batches at a time, until smooth. Add season and place aside to cool until just warm.

5. Divide the soup between bowls, season and top with dollops of fresh dill sprigs and low-fat plain yogurt.

Carrot Lentil Soup

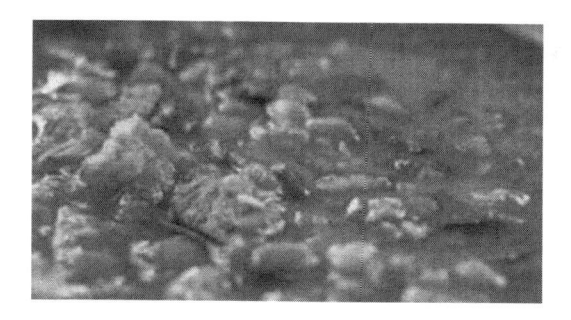

Cooking Minutes: *30 minutes*

Preparation Time: *10 minutes*

Calorie count: *191 Calories*

Makes 2 Servings

Ingredients:

½ cup (118 grams) Green/Brown Lentils, rinsed and sorted through

7 ounces (200 grams) canned crushed Tomatoes

1½ cups (360 ml) Fat-Free, low sodium Vegetable Broth

1 teaspoon Flora Cooking Spray

½ cup (118 grams) Onion, diced

½ cup (118 grams) Carrots, diced

¼ cup (59 grams) Celery, chopped

Salt and Pepper to taste

Directions:

1. In a Dutch oven heat Flora Cooking Spray on medium heat. Gently sauté onions, celery and carrots until softened. Stir into vegetables.

2. Add lentils, tomatoes and low sodium vegetable broth. Bring to boiling point, then lower the heat and allow to simmer for 25 minutes.

3. Add salt and pepper to taste if necessary.

Quick & Easy Asparagus and Salmon

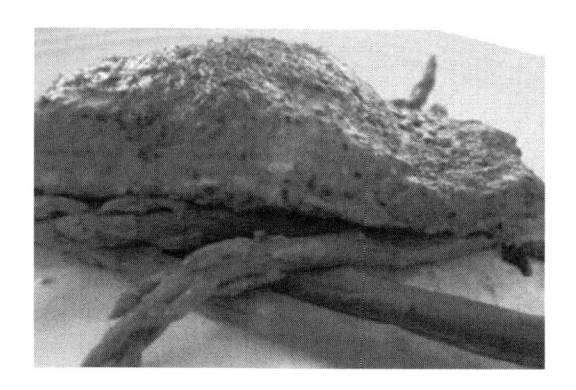

Cooking Minutes: *12-15 minutes*

Preparation Time: *10 minutes*

Calorie count: *235 Calories*

Makes 2 Servings

Ingredients:

½ pound (226 grams) Fresh Asparagus Spears, cut into 2-inch pieces

¾ teaspoons (4.5 ml) Extra Virgin Olive Oil

½ pound (226 grams) Salmon Fillets with skin, Fresh or Frozen

½ teaspoon Lemon Peel, finely shredded

½ teaspoon fresh parsley, trimmed

Unrefined sea salt and freshly ground pepper according to taste

Directions:

1. Preheat oven to 450 degrees Fahrenheit. Place two (1 large and 1 medium) cast-iron skillet or oven-safe heavy skillet in oven.

2. In a medium bowl combine asparagus and ½ teaspoon olive oil; sprinkle with salt and pepper to taste. Brush with the remaining olive oil on both sides of fish; sprinkle lightly with salt and pepper.

3. Carefully remove both skillets from the oven. Put the fish with the skin side down, in the large size skillet. Put the asparagus in medium size skillet. Return both skillets to oven. Allow to bake for about 12 minutes, or until when the fish flakes easily if tested with a fork and asparagus is crisp-tender.

4. To serve, sprinkle fish with lemon peel and parsley.

Flavourful Lemon Grilled Chicken Breast

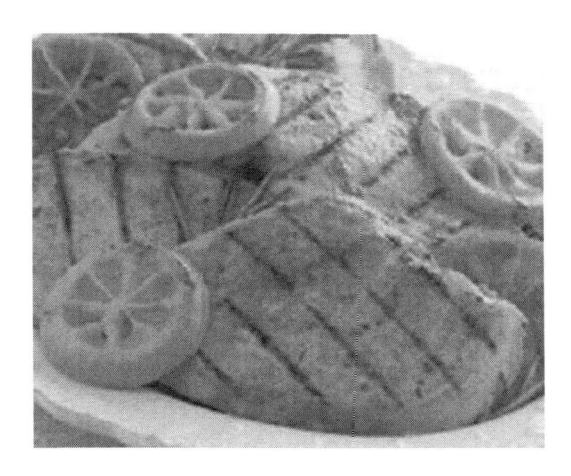

Cooking Minutes: *12-15 minutes*

Preparation Time: *1 hour 20 minutes*

Calorie count: *161 Calories*

Makes 2 Servings

Ingredients:

2 Chicken Breast, halves skinless, boneless (about 12 oz./85g in total)

½ tablespoon Fresh Lemon Thyme or Thyme, finely trimmed

1/8 teaspoon Ground Black Pepper

1 lemon, halved or sliced (optional)

¼ cup (60 ml) reduced-sodium Chicken Broth

½ tablespoon lemon peel (zest), finely shredded

1 tablespoon (15 ml) Lemon Juice

Fresh Lemon Thyme or Thyme Sprigs (optional)

Directions:

1. In a shallow bowl Place the chicken breasts in a re-sealable plastic bag. For marinade, in a small bowl stir together reduced-sodium chicken broth, lemon zest and juice, 1 tablespoon thyme and pepper to taste. Pour the chicken broth sauce over the chicken. Seal the plastic bag.
2. Marinate in the refrigerator for about 2 hours while turning the bag at intervals. Drain the chicken, and reserve the marinade for afterwards.
3. Grill chicken on the rack of an uncovered grill directly over medium coals for 12 to 15 minutes or until no longer pink at about 170 degrees Fahrenheit, turning and brushing with marinade halfway through grilling.
4. Discard leftover marinade. When the last 3 minutes of grilling is left, add in the lemon halves to the grill.
5. Serve the grilled chicken with the grilled lemons. You may top with more thyme if desired.

Tasty Grilled Sea Bass

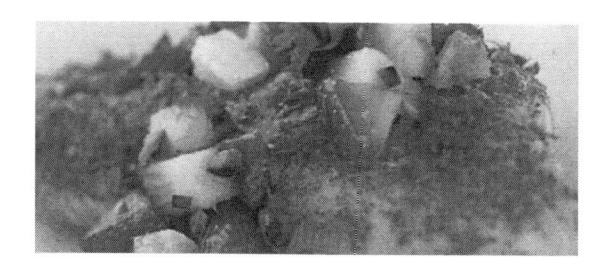

Cooking Minutes: *17 to 18 minutes*

Preparation Time: *20 minutes*

Calorie count: *130 Calories*

Makes 2 Servings

Ingredients:

2 Sea Bass or Halibut Steaks, fresh or frozen, 1 inch thick (thawed, rinsed and pat dry)

1/8 cup Seeded Fresh chili Pepper, (about ½ of a small) finely chopped

1 tablespoon Fresh Cilantro, snipped

¼ teaspoon cumin seeds, toasted*

Salt to taste

½ of a small Lime (finely shred lime peel then peel, section, and chop lime)

1/8 teaspoon Cayenne Pepper

½ cup (118 grams) Fresh Strawberries, chopped

Directions:

1. In a small bowl combine lime peel, the cayenne pepper and the ¼ teaspoon salt. Evenly distribute this mixture over each side of the fish steaks; rub in with your fingers.

2. Arrange medium-hot coals around a drip pan. Check for medium heat above pan. Afterwards, put the fish on the greased grill rack over the drip pan. Next, cover and grill for about 8 minutes for each ½-inch thickness or until fish flakes easily when checked with a fork. Carefully turn once you have reached half of the grilling time.

3. Meanwhile, in a medium bowl combine chopped lime, cilantro, strawberries, cumin seeds, chili pepper and the a little salt (about 1/8 teaspoon). Serve with the grilled fish.

Tip:

*For toasting cumin seeds, in a small skillet heat cumin seeds over medium heat until fragrant, shaking skillet occasionally.

Chicken Salad

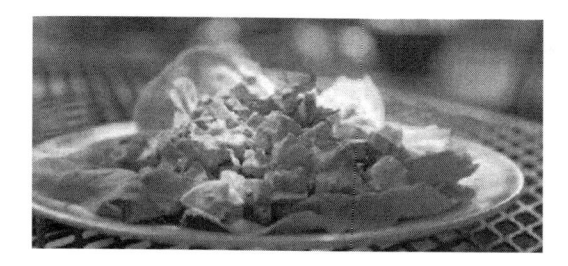

Preparation Time: *5 to 8 minutes*

Calorie count: *89 Calories*

Makes 2 Servings

Ingredients:

½ cup (118 grams)Cooked Chicken Breast, diced

1 Stuffed Olive, chopped fine (optional)

2 Lettuce Leaves

2 tablespoon Low Fat Mayonnaise

1/8 teaspoon Apple Cider Vinegar

1 tablespoons Olive Oil

1/8 cup Celery, diced

Directions:
Place all ingredients, except lettuce, in a large bowl. Add mayonnaise and toss. Serve on lettuce leaves.

You Can Do It!

You've proved that you've taken responsibility for your own health, and consequently, you've made a courageous step towards your health goals by purchasing this book. It is true that we'll never get anywhere unless we start somewhere. With that being said, now that you've embarked on a weight loss journey, it is essential that you use these recipes in order to get the results. The ball is in your court. You can turn things around and obtain an ideal weight using these fast diet recipes. If others have done it, you can do it too.

Remember that if we are serious about losing weight, consistency becomes very important. I encourage you to stick with the program in order to really realize the benefits. With the recipes in this book, you will always have control over your weight and your overall health. Even if you drift off a bit from this fast diet and gain unwanted weight, years from now you will still be equipped with the recipes in this book. As a result, you will be able to turn your situation around whenever you want to. We should never forget that our dreams cannot be realized without good health; therefore staying healthy is our best option.

In the end, losing weight can be as easy or as hard as you make it. Start using these recipes and lose weight on the fast diet.

All the best and happy fasting,
Gillian

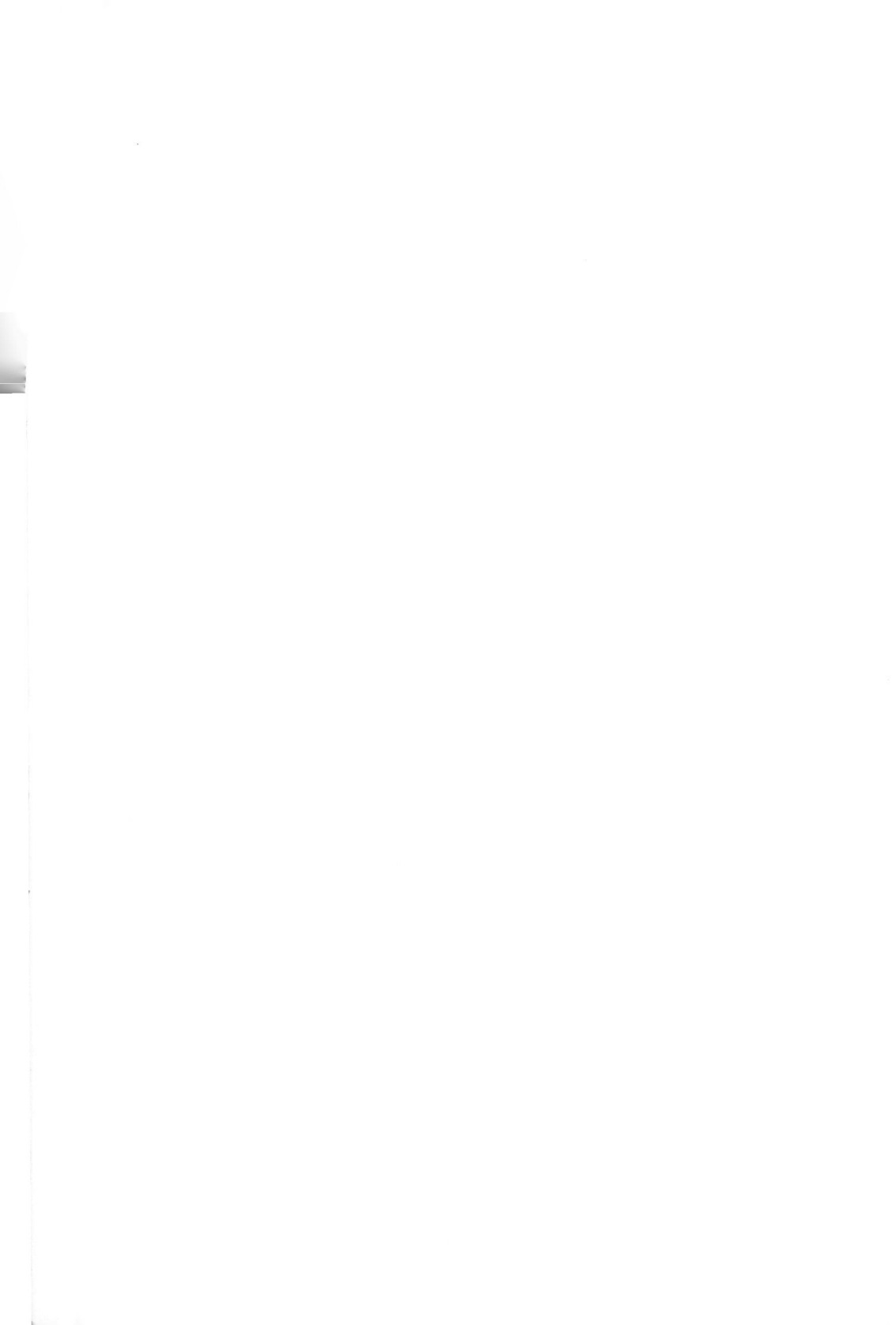

Printed in Great Britain
by Amazon.co.uk, Ltd.,
Marston Gate.